FATTY LIVER: Causes and abstaining from fatty liver (Disease) both adults and children.

William George E.

Table of contents

Chapter 1

What is fatty liver

Fat in the liver normally accumulates when a person eats more fat and sugar than his or her body can tolerate. This is more frequent in those who are overweight or obese but may also occur in adults with appropriate body weights. If fat accumulates in the liver to more than 5% of its total volume, the liver is said to be "fatty." Although having this issue may not cause any immediate damage, there is a fear that additional fat in the liver can render the organ prone to subsequent injuries such as inflammation and scarring.

What Parents Should Know About Kids and Fatty Liver Disease

Nonalcoholic fatty liver disease, a disorder typically linked with obesity, affects an estimated 80 million individuals in the United States and is the most prevalent chronic liver ailment in children and adolescents. We talked with pediatric gastroenterologist Jennifer Woo Baidal, MD, MPH, about causes for this development, possible health repercussions, and treatments to avoid or reverse the illness in children.

What is fatty liver disease, and what do parents need to know about it?

Fatty liver disease arises when too much fat accumulates in the liver and starts an inflammatory process that injures liver cells. It's often symptomless, but as it worsens, fatty liver disease may interfere with important liver processes.

With the growth in childhood obesity, more kids are acquiring the condition, and we're seeing more in our clinic. Many parents are aware that obesity may lead to type 2 diabetes and other significant metabolic diseases, but there is considerably less understanding of the relationship between obesity and liver disease.

There are also certain genetic variations that may raise the risk, with or without fat.

How many kids have fatty liver disease, and what is the health impact?

We identify it by detecting blood levels of an enzyme called ALT, which is a sign of liver damage. But it's difficult to detect the inflammatory component without a liver biopsy, so the prevalence figures are erroneous. Autopsy studies reveal that roughly 1 in 10 children and adolescents have fatty livers, with or without inflammation.

In adults, the condition is a growing cause of liver transplantation and, in some cases, liver cancer.

Cirrhosis—scarring of the liver owing to persistent inflammation—is uncommon in youngsters, but it's a worrying long-term consequence that may lead to end-stage liver disease. I've seen a youngster as young as 6 with inflammation and an adolescent with cirrhosis.

The liver manufactures numerous proteins, regulates the body's metabolism, and filters out poisons from our blood. If it stops functioning, a liver transplant is the only option.

At what age does fatty liver disease become an issue?

Previous research has focused on fatty liver in adolescents and young adults; thus, we recently
looked at younger children (link is external and opens in a new window). We observed that 3-year-olds with a larger waist circumference had higher levels of ALT—a marker for liver damage—by the time they were 8.

Those with bigger increases in waist circumference and other indicators of obesity also had higher ALT levels in mid-childhood. This suggests that we need to intervene early in a child's life to avoid excess weight gain and consequent liver inflammation.

Besides lowering weight, can anything else prevent or treat nonalcoholic fatty liver disease?

Maintaining a healthy weight by eating fewer processed foods and exercising frequently is the major approach for adolescents and adults to avoid nonalcoholic fatty liver disease.

There may possibly be a function for vitamin E. We've been examining a kind of vitamin E, D-alpha tocopherol, that is used to minimize liver inflammation and damage in children and adults with fatty liver disease.

We'd want to know whether vitamin E can also reduce inflammation in youngsters who are at risk for fatty liver disease.

Recently (this link is external and opens in a new window), we identified an association between alpha-tocopherol and
ALT in young infants of all weight categories: Those with decreased dietary intake of alpha tocopherol—the beneficial sort of vitamin E—had higher ALT levels in mid-childhood. This shows that ingesting prescribed levels of vitamin E—an antioxidant—may reduce liver inflammation. Foods that are high in vitamin E include spinach, tomatoes, avocados, various kinds of seafood, and nuts and seeds.

Vitamin E from supplements is absorbed differently than the food

version, so it's uncertain whether supplements may reduce liver inflammation. That's a research project we want to initiate, but we first need a noninvasive diagnostic that is more specific than ALT and less
invasive than a liver biopsy to identify at-risk youngsters.

Should children be checked for fatty liver disease?

Screening efforts are inconsistent, in part because there is no therapy other than weight reduction and we don't have a great noninvasive screening instrument. Some physicians assess ALT levels in all obese children beginning at about age 10. But as our research reveals, we urgently need new approaches to screen, diagnose, and treat fatty liver, beginning in infancy.

Chapter 2

Causes of fatty liver

The most prevalent cause of fatty liver disease in Canada is obesity. In 2018, approximately 30% of Canadians aged 18 and up (roughly 7.3 million people) reported height and weight that classified them as overweight or obese.

Besides obesity, dietary factors of fatty liver disease are:

Starvation and protein malnutrition Long-term use of complete parenteral nutrition (a feeding treatment that includes pumping nutrients straight into the circulation) (a feeding procedure that involves infusing

nutrients directly into the bloodstream)
Intestinal bypass surgery for obesity
Rapid weight loss
Certain disorders typically accompany and may contribute to fatty liver disease:

Diabetes mellitus
Hyperlipidemia (elevated lipids in the blood) (elevated lipids in the blood)
Insulin resistance and high blood pressure
Other factors include:

Genetic factors\sDrugs and chemicals.

Can children acquire fatty liver disease?
Fatty liver disease is already becoming obvious in youngsters,

owing in large part to an alarming rise in juvenile obesity. Currently:

It is believed that one Canadian kid in 10 is overweight, a statistic that has roughly quadrupled in the previous decade.
In Canada, fatty liver disease is believed to occur in one in five overweight or obese children.
Fatty liver disease affects roughly 3% of children and 25–55% of obese youngsters.
Fatty liver disease may be detected in children as early as two years of age.

Fatty liver disease may also arise in children with healthy body weights but who may have bigger waist circumferences than other children of the same weight and height.
Fatty liver disease is more frequent in males than girls and tends to arise in

youngsters of Caucasian or South Asian heritage.
Fatty liver disease is more likely in children who have family members with fatty livers or type 2 diabetes.

The etiology of fatty liver disease is considered to be connected to variables such as diets rich in fatty foods and simple carbohydrates and sedentary lifestyles, especially in children or adolescents who are overweight or obese.

In children, a fatty liver may be caused by a range of conditions including those linked to difficulties with copper metabolism (e.g., Wilson Disease), viral hepatitis, or a variety of autoimmune diseases. It is vitally crucial that your doctor makes sure that your kid does not have these problems initially.

NAFLD can only be diagnosed in children when all other probable causes of fatty liver have been ruled out. If your doctor or healthcare provider believes your kid may be at risk for NAFLD, they may request certain blood tests and an ultrasound of the abdomen to establish if your child has NAFLD or not. Consult your doctor about what sorts of testing your kid has to take to discover whether your child has NAFLD.

When it comes to youngsters, measuring waist circumference and your kid's height may help you decide whether your child is accumulating additional fat around the center of their body. It is crucial to measure your child's waist circumference, in the same method, each time it is done.

The specific figure that you obtain for a kid's waist circumference is not what is crucial, since each child develops at various rates and therefore each child may have a different number. A common rule of thumb is to measure the ratio between your child's waist circumference and their height (in centimeters) (in centimeters). A ratio larger than 0.5 may imply that the youngster is depositing a little excess fat around their belly. However, it does NOT indicate your kid has NAFLD.

Waist-to-height ratio = WC (cm) (cm)

Healthy Body Weights for Children
The greatest method to assess whether your child's body weight is in the healthy range is to plot your child's weight and body mass index (BMI) on growth curves. A healthy

body weight is when your child's weight or BMI falls between the third percentile and the 95th percentile.

If your kid's BMI is over the 95th percentile then your youngster is obese. If your child's BMI is between the 85th percentile and 95th percentile, they may be overweight.

It is vital to watch the 'trend' of where your kid is 'tracking' on the development curve and not just one moment in time. Remember your kid is growing and therefore you can anticipate that your child's BMI will alter with time.

BMI is computed precisely like adults. Your child's weight (in kg) divided by your child's height (in meters) squared

Chapter 3

Symptoms and discovering of fatty liver in earlier stage

Many people recognize heavy drinking may cause liver disease, but not everyone realizes a fatty diet by itself can also harm the liver in both adults and children. Fatty liver disease symptoms not attributable to alcohol usage are extremely similar to those of alcoholic liver disease and may cause similarly serious liver damage.

Left untreated, nonalcoholic fatty liver disease (NAFLD) may proceed to the more dangerous disorder

nonalcoholic steatohepatitis (NASH) and potentially complete liver failure. Unfortunately, NAFLD seldom presents signs until it's severe. Learn the signs and symptoms that might suggest fatty liver disease—and when to consult a doctor.

Ache in the Upper-Right Abdomen\sman with stomach pain gripping stomach with hands.

The liver is the body's biggest important organ; it occupies space beneath the bottom section of the right rib cage. One of the rare indications of fatty liver disease, particularly in youngsters, is discomfort in this approximate location, generally in the upper-right quadrant of the abdomen, just below the rib cage.

The pain arises when fatty liver disease advances to inflammation and expansion of the organ (NASH), which strains the capsule (the liver's covering) to produce discomfort. However, numerous illnesses may produce pain in the same location, including appendicitis and gallstones, so visit a healthcare expert to investigate this symptom.

Unexplained Wearines.
Tiredness may be the most prevalent symptom reported to clinicians. Unexplained fatigue may be indicative of hundreds of illnesses and, as a sign of fatty liver disease in adults, exhaustion again joins the list. Your doctor likely will first try to rule out simpler explanations for fatigue before progressing to a diagnosis of fatty liver disease, unless you exhibit other symptoms like right upper-quadrant pain, or if you're at

high risk for fatty liver disease due to obesity, high cholesterol, family history, or heavy drinking.

Elevated Liver Enzymes\doctor holding liver function test result indicating bilirubin level
Whether you have type 2 diabetes, metabolic syndrome, or another illness linked with fatty liver disease, your doctor may do a blood test to establish if you have NAFLD—even if you don't have symptoms. Elevated levels of the enzymes aminotransferase (ALT) and aspartate aminotransferase (AST) suggest liver malfunction of some type, which might be caused by fatty liver disease. Your healthcare practitioner will assess these test findings in conjunction with your personal history, present physical state, risk factors and the results of

other tests before establishing a diagnosis of NAFLD or fatty liver disease attributable to alcohol.

Visible Fat in the Liver\doctor-looking-at-liver-scan Imaging procedures like ultrasound and MRI may provide images that demonstrate if fatty deposits exist in your liver. Fatty accumulation in the liver is a clear-cut symptom of fatty liver disease. But imaging techniques can't identify the existence of inflammation or the formation of scar tissue, which indicate how far the illness has gone. For that your doctor may need to acquire a tissue sample (biopsy) (biopsy).

Liver Inflammation and Fibrosis\sconcept artwork of obese

guy with fatty liver, displaying inset of microscopic liver damage

As nonalcoholic fatty liver disease worsens, it may lead to liver enlargement, inflammation and fibrosis (scar tissue production) (scar tissue development). This is nonalcoholic steatohepatitis (NASH) (NASH).

To diagnose NASH, physicians biopsy the liver. The presence of inflammation or scar tissue in the sample implies NASH. If you have been diagnosed with NAFLD, you may lower your chance of NASH by decreasing weight, eating a heart-healthy diet, and exercising frequently to maintain your liver operating as well as possible.

Chapter 4

The perfect diet for fatty liver patient

10 Foods to Include in a Healthy Liver Diet.

Non-alcoholic fatty liver disease (NAFLD) is one of the most prevalent

causes of liver disease in the United States. It's a condition in which excess fat is stored in the liver and may lead to cirrhosis and liver failure if left untreated.

NAFLD is more prevalent in people who are living with particular conditions such as obesity and type 2 diabetes, and unlike alcohol-related liver disease, NAFLD is not caused by heavy alcohol intake.

In a healthy body, the liver removes toxins and generates bile, a protein that breaks down fat into fatty acids so that they may be absorbed. Fatty liver disease damages the liver and impairs its ability to function properly, but lifestyle changes may prevent it from worsening.

The main line of treatment for NAFLD is weight reduction, employing a

combination of calorie restriction, exercise, and excellent nutrition.
In general, the diet for fatty liver disease includes the following:

fruits and vegetables; high-fiber plants, including legumes and whole grains; significantly limiting consumption of specific meals and drinks, including those heavy in added sugar, salt, processed carbs, and saturated fat; no alcohol.
The quantity of weight that you should drop to treat NAFLD will depend on the amount of additional body fat that you have.

Your healthcare team may help you decide on a suitable weight loss objective based on your overall health. Trusted sources frequently recommend a nutrient-dense, whole-foods-based diet rich in fiber,

protein, and unsaturated fats for people with NAFLD.
Here are a few items to put in your healthy liver diet:

1. Coffee to help lower abnormal liver enzymes
Your regular cup of coffee could help protect your liver from NAFLD.

A trusted source revealed that regular coffee consumption is related to a lower likelihood of developing NAFLD as well as a decreased risk of the development of liver fibrosis in those already diagnosed with NAFLD.
Caffeine also appears to reduce the number of abnormal liver enzymes in people who are predisposed to liver disease.

2. Greens to prevent fat buildup

Compounds included in spinach and other leafy greens may help battle fatty liver disease.

A trusted source also revealed that eating spinach notably lowered the risk of NAFLD, possibly due to the nitrate and unique polyphenols present in the leafy green. Interestingly enough, the study focused on raw spinach, whereas cooked spinach did not offer the same dramatic advantages. This could be because cooking spinach (and other leafy greens) may result in reduced polyphenolic content and antioxidant activity.

3. Beans and soy to minimize the risk of NAFLD

Both beans and soy have exhibited potential when it comes to minimizing the risk of NAFLD.

A scientific overview
Trusted Source on Diet and Liver Disease points out that legumes such as lentils, chickpeas, soybeans, and peas are not only nutritionally dense meals, but also have resistant starches that help increase gut health. Bean consumption may even help obese people lower their blood glucose and cholesterol levels.Furthermore, a 2019 study found that diets high in legumes significantly reduced the risk of NFALD.

Noted for its ability to help lower triglyceride levels and possibly protect against visceral fat buildup.

Additionally, tofu is a low-fat meal that functions as a respectable source of protein, making it a wonderful alternative if you're seeking to minimize your fat consumption.

4. Fish to decrease inflammation and fat levels

Fatty fish such as salmon, sardines, tuna, and trout are high in omega-3 fatty acids. Research from a trusted source shows that supplementation with omega-3s may benefit individuals with NAFLD by reducing liver fat, boosting protective HDL cholesterol, and lowering triglyceride levels.

5. Oatmeal for fiber

Whole-grain, fiber-rich diets like oatmeal are associated with a decreased incidence of NAFLD-related diseases.

According to research (Trusted Source), a healthy diet rich in high-fiber foods like oats can help patients with NAFLD lower their triglyceride levels.

6. Nuts to aid in decreasing inflammation

A diet high in nuts is connected with reduced inflammation, insulin resistance, oxidative stress, and a lower prevalence of NAFLD.

A big research

Trusted Source from China found that increased nut consumption was strongly related to a lower prevalence of NAFLD, and in its research, Trusted Source has noticed that patients with fatty liver disease who eat walnuts have improved liver function tests.

7. Turmeric to decrease signs of liver damage

High doses of curcumin, the active component in turmeric, might lessen indications of liver damage in people with NAFLD.

Studies

According to a trusted source specializing in turmeric supplements, the bright orange root may lower levels of blood alanine aminotransferase (ALT) and aspartate aminotransferase (AST), two enzymes that are significantly elevated in people with fatty liver disease.

8. Sunflower seeds for antioxidants

Sunflower seeds are extremely plentiful in vitamin E, an antioxidant commonly used (via supplementation) in the treatment of NAFLD.

While most research involving NAFLD and vitamin E concentrates on supplements, a 100-gram serving of sunflower seeds delivers around 20 milligrams of this trusted source of vitamin E, more than 100 percent of the daily recommended value.

Trusted Source If you're seeking to enhance your vitamin E consumption naturally, sunflower seeds are a wonderful starting place.

9. Increase unsaturated fat intake.

Swapping out sources of saturated fat—like butter, fatty cuts of meat, sausages, and cured meats—for unsaturated fat sources—like avocados, olive oil, nut butter, and fatty fish—may be helpful for individuals with NAFLD.

Because of its emphasis on foods high in unsaturated fat and its potential to lower total cholesterol, the Mediterranean diet is sometimes recommended for people with NAFLD.

10. Garlic to boost overall health

This vegetable not only adds flavor to meals, but a small scientific study also revealed that garlic powder supplements (Trusted Source) may assist in lowering body weight and fat in folks with fatty liver disease.

In a recent 2020 study (Trusted Source), patients with NAFLD who took 800 mg of garlic powder every day for 15 weeks revealed reductions in liver fat and improved enzyme levels.

When it comes to whole food consumption, a 2019 study

Trusted Source found that frequent ingestion of raw garlic was inversely connected with NAFLD in Chinese males (but not women) (but not women).

6 types of foods to avoid if you have fatty liver disease

If you have fatty liver disease, your doctor may suggest avoiding certain foods or at least eating them sparingly. These foods typically lead to weight gain and may elevate blood sugar.

Avoid as much as possible.

Alcohol.
Alcohol may be a key cause of fatty liver disease as well as other liver illnesses.
Added sugar. Stay away from sugary foods such as sweets, cookies, sodas, and fruit juices. High blood sugar increases the amount of fat deposition in the liver.

Fried foods.
These are high in fat and calories.
Add salt. Consuming too much salt might raise the risk of NAFLD. It's recommended by Trusted Source to reduce salt consumption to fewer

than 2,300 mg per day. People who have high blood pressure should restrict salt consumption to no more than 1,500 mg per day.

White bread, rice, and pasta White flour is often highly processed, and things prepared from it might elevate your blood sugar more than whole grains, owing to a lack of fiber.

Red meat.
Beef and deli meats are high in saturated fat.

What does a diet plan for fatty liver disease look like?

If you've been diagnosed with fatty liver disease, your doctor may advise working with a nutritionist to come up with a meal plan. Here's what a typical everyday lunch may look like:

Meal Menu\breakfast

Hot oatmeal combined with 2 teaspoons. almond butter, 1 teaspoon. chia seeds, and 1 cup mixed berries; • 1 cup black coffee tea; •

 lunch or green tea\slunch • Salad of spinach with a balsamic vinegar and olive oil dressing
grilled chicken; • 1 small baked potato; •
1 cup boiling broccoli, carrots, or other vegetables; Snack• 1 tbsp. peanut butter on sliced apples or 2 teaspoons. hummus with raw veggies.

Dinner:
A small mixed-bean salad; • 3 oz. grilled salmon; • 1 cup cooked broccoli; • 1 cup cooked quinoa; • 1 cup mixed berries.

Chapter 5

Best sports for fatty liver patient

How to Exercise if You Have a Liver DiseaseExercise for liver disease What is included in this article?
How exercise helps liver healthTypes of exercise: frequency and perseverance.
How exercise helps liver healthRegular exercise and a good diet are the best strategies to not only maintain a healthy liver but also a healthy weight and immune system. According to LiveStrong, exercise can help with liver disease in a variety of ways.First, it helps you regulate your

weight by burning extra fat, which may prevent obesity. Exercise may also help improve levels of "good" high-density lipoprotein cholesterol, which in turn decreases your triglyceride levels and "bad" low-density lipoprotein cholesterol. Exercise also helps prevent and treat other illnesses related to fatty liver disease, such as type 2 diabetes.

Types of exercise
Weight-bearing exercise strengthens your bones, which is particularly important since liver illness may induce osteoporosis, especially in women.Yoga may be less stressful on the body, stimulate blood flow, and improve bones and muscles.

Aerobic activity such as cycling, jogging, or aggressively walking outdoors is fantastic for your cardiovascular system and has an influence on blood oxygenation. Aerobic exercise boosts your heart rate and increases the quantity of oxygen that flows to your organs, including the liver.

FrequencyLiver illness may frequently produce weariness, so it is vital to consider this when establishing plans and goals for yourself. Do not push yourself too hard and begin exercising gradually. Dr. Melissa Palmer, author and practicing hepatologist, suggests exercising three times a week to start out with and aiming for 30-45 minutes; anything more is a bonus.

Talk to your doctor or physician about how frequently it would suit you, and remember to start small and work your way up to more since doing too much too soon might cause harm.

PerseveranceOne week of exercise will not show you any physical improvements; it is crucial to remember that you will need to figure in exercise as part of your weekly routine from now on. You will experience favorable mental and physical gains as time goes on, and exercising should become simpler for you.

Remember that being healthy is not a destination; it is a continuing journey, and your lifestyle modifications should be lasting.

Getting motivated might be challenging, particularly if you are not accustomed to exercise. Try these strategies for becoming motivated:

Monitor your mood: Write down how you feel after you work out; similarly, write down how you feel when you miss an exercise. We know which one will make you feel better.Wear your training clothing.

This should encourage you to want to work out. Nobody likes to take their workout clothes off without having exercised.Keep your eyes on the prize—remember why you're exercising, whether it's to lose weight, get in shape, or improve your mood.Join a group: Joining an exercise group means you will have lots of other individuals who are driven and who will keep you motivated too.Commit to a class: If you pay for a class, then you have the extra motivation to attend. Losing money and not working out is far worse than simply missing the exercise!

Exercising on a budgetYou absolutely do not need a pricey gym membership to start exercising. Running and brisk walking are excellent ways to get started, and some parks and beaches even have fitness equipment available for free use.There are many free videos on YouTube that can provide you with endless possibilities for a good workout in the comfort of your own home.

There may also be lessons in your region that simply require a contribution; check local Facebook groups and notice boards for additional information.

Staying hydratedEnsure that you keep hydrated when exercising or performing sports; hydration is a critical component of liver health. When we work out, we sweat more, which might lead to dehydration if we are not consuming enough water.

This may create various difficulties for the body. If you struggle to remain hydrated, sign up for our Kitchen Companion for seven suggestions on staying hydrated. If this book is helpful, recommend it to your loved ones.

9 798366 345460